Olga Vysogortseva

Physiotherapy and physical therapy in the rehabilitation of children with DST

Olga Vysogortseva

Physiotherapy and physical therapy in the rehabilitation of children with DST

ScienciaScripts

Imprint

Any brand names and product names mentioned in this book are subject to trademark, brand or patent protection and are trademarks or registered trademarks of their respective holders. The use of brand names, product names, common names, trade names, product descriptions etc. even without a particular marking in this work is in no way to be construed to mean that such names may be regarded as unrestricted in respect of trademark and brand protection legislation and could thus be used by anyone.

Cover image: www.ingimage.com

This book is a translation from the original published under ISBN 978-620-2-19916-2.

Publisher:
Sciencia Scripts
is a trademark of
Dodo Books Indian Ocean Ltd. and OmniScriptum S.R.L publishing group

120 High Road, East Finchley, London, N2 9ED, United Kingdom
Str. Armeneasca 28/1, office 1, Chisinau MD-2012, Republic of Moldova, Europe
Managing Directors: Ieva Konstantinova, Victoria Ursu
info@omniscriptum.com

Printed at: see last page
ISBN: 978-620-8-05689-6

Table of Contents

INTRODUCTION

Physical development is the most important indicator of children's health [54]. Negative trends in the physical development of children and adolescents may be due to the deterioration of the environmental situation, including anthropogenic loads, the presence of iodine deficiency, a decrease in the quality of nutrition, an increase in stressful situations in the daily life of children, deterioration of somatic health [2,43] and other factors. One of the factors that worsen children's health and affect their physical development is connective tissue dysplasia (CTD) [43].

The problem of DST has recently aroused great interest of medical practitioners due to the increased detection of patients with this pathology [34,43], their early disability, shortening of life, and death at working age.

DST is now considered as the constitutional basis of multi-organ disorders in children and adolescents[4,25].

The presence of dysplastic-dependent cosmetic changes combined with asthenia form psychological features of these patients: low mood, loss of pleasure and interest in activities, emotional lability, pessimistic assessment of the future, often with self-injurious and suicidal thoughts. A natural consequence of psychological distress is the limitation of social activity, deterioration of the quality of life and a significant decrease in social adaptation, most relevant in adolescence and young adulthood [4,25,34].

The degree of dysplasia severity predetermines the frequency and time of irreversible disabling consequences of connective tissue remodeling, necessitating the development of timely and modern therapeutic and preventive measures for this category of children and adolescents [25,34].

The management of patients with DST is an open question. To date, there are no universally recognized approaches to the treatment of patients with DST. Given that gene therapy is currently unavailable to medicine, the physician should use any means that will help to stop the progression of the disease. The leading component of therapy of patients with DST should be non-medicamentous effects (therapeutic exercise, dosed loads, aerobic regimen). [17,34]. However, often a significant factor limiting the achievement of the target level of physical activity in patients with DST is poor subjective tolerance to exercise (abundance of asthenic, vegetative complaints, episodes of hypotension), which reduces patients' adherence to this type of rehabilitation measures. [17]. All the above-mentioned factors determined the relevance of our study.

3

Chapter I. Concept of connective tissue dysplasia (CTD)

General information about the structure of connective tissue

In the process of embryonic development of an organism from the middle germinal leaflet (mesoderm) develops the so-called germinal tissue - mesenchyme, from which two rudiments are further differentiated. One of them gives connective tissue, including bones, cartilage and smooth muscles. Thus, many tissues and organs that have little in common when viewed superficially appear to be embryologically related. Moreover, this intrinsic relatedness may be manifested by identical lesions and responses under pathologic conditions [1,3]. Connective tissue in the human body is the most diverse. It includes such dissimilar substances as bone and fat, skin and blood. Therefore, it is customary to speak of a group of connective tissues. (A) Connective tissue proper. 1. The loose beginning of the development of blood and blood vessels, the other is the formation of all kinds of connective tissue (accompanies all vessels, i.e., is almost everywhere). 2. Dense connective tissue: unformed (skin) and formed (tendons, ligaments, aponeuroses, dura mater, etc.). 3. Adipose tissue (skin, omentum, mesentery, etc.). 4. Reticular tissue (red bone marrow, lymph nodes, thymus, spleen). 5. Pigmented tissue (hair, retina of eyeball, tanned skin, etc.). (B) Cartilage tissue. 1. Hyaline cartilage (connection of ribs to sternum, cartilage in larynx, trachea, etc.). 2. Elastic cartilage (ear lobe, larynx). 3. Fibrous cartilage (intervertebral discs, pubic symphysis). (C) Bone tissue. (D) Blood. The named tissues are united not only by common origin, but also by common structure and function [17,18,19]. Any tissue consists of cells (nervous, epithelial, muscular), but what is characteristic is that only connective tissue has intercellular substance between these cells. The main structural elements of connective tissue are. (A)

Cellular elements: 1. Fibroblasts and their varieties - osteoblasts, chondroblasts, odontoblasts. 2. Macrophages (histiocytes). 3. Mast cells (labrocytes). (B) Extracellular matrix: 1. Fibers: collagen (15 types) and elastin. 2. Amorphous matter: glycosaminoglycans and proteoglycans. The content of the amorphous component determines the consistency of connective tissue. Collagen fibers give the whole tissue strength and allow it to stretch, and elastic fibers return the tissue to its original position after it is stretched. The functions of connective tissue are biomechanical, trophic, barrier, plastic, and morphogenetic [16,17,18,19].

Current understanding of connective tissue dysplasia

Connective tissue dysplasia (DCT) (dis - disorder, plasia - development, formation) is a disorder of connective tissue development in the embryonic and postnatal periods, a genetically determined condition characterized by defects in fibrous structures and the basic substance of connective tissue, leading to homeostasis disorders at tissue, organ and organismal levels in the form of various morphofunctional disorders of visceral and locomotor organs with a progressive course, determining the features of associated pathology [1,2,3,20,33,34,34,35,36].

DST is a genetically determined process, i.e. mutations in the genes responsible for fiber synthesis are at the root of everything. As a result of mutations, collagen chains are not formed correctly. They are shorter (deletion), or longer (insertion), or they include the wrong amino acid (point mutation). So-called abnormal collagen trimers are obtained, which cannot withstand proper mechanical loads [33,35,36,44,45,46,61,62].

Epidemiologic data on the prevalence of DST itself are controversial due to different classification and diagnostic approaches. The prevalence of individual DST features varies by age and sex. According to the most modest data, the prevalence of DST at least correlates with the prevalence of major socially significant non-infectious diseases [3,14,15,33,34,35].The frequency of DST syndrome detection is quite high, ranging from 26 to 80% depending on the study group [8,9,18]. Thus, according to G. I. Nechaeva et al. (1997), 74 to 85% of school-age children have various signs of DST [33,34,35].

In the 1990s of the last century, a **classification** was adopted, according to which two groups of ST pathology were also distinguished. The first group includes differentiated DSTs with a certain type of inheritance, more often autosomal dominant, and clearly defined clinical symptoms: Marfan syndrome, Ehlers-Danlos syndrome, osteogenesis imperfecta, etc., which are rare and belong to collagenopathies [10,25,26,27,28,29]. In particular, the current criteria for the diagnosis of Marfan syndrome (Ghent Diagnostic Nosology) were developed in 1996 [38]. The second group includes undifferentiated connective tissue dysplasias (NDCT), which are distinguished as a nosologically independent DST syndrome of polygenic multifactorial nature, manifested by external phenotypic features with dysplastic changes in the NT and clinically significant dysfunction of one or more internal organs [8,9,10,11].

Diagnosis of undifferentiated connective tissue dysplasia is based on the following symptoms and additional data (anthropometry, external respiration, reduced heart size, reduced blood pressure, plethysmography, specific characteristics of electrocardiography and ultrasound phleboscanning) [40,41,42,62,63]. Certain phenotypic or external features allow us to suspect connective tissue dysplasia syndrome already at the stage of physical examination. Clinical examination of the relatives of patients with such diseases does not reveal typical signs of connective tissue lesions, whereas the data of pedigrees testify to the "accumulation" in the families of patients of such pathologies as osteochondrosis, osteoarthritis, joint hypermobility, varicose veins, hemorrhoids, vision pathology, flat feet, tendency to bleeding, etc. [21,22,23,24]. [21,22,23,24]. The manifestations of DST include not only specific appearance and cosmetic defects, but also severe pathologic changes in internal organs and musculoskeletal system.

The clinical and morphologic manifestations of DST include:

• Skeletal changes: asthenic physique, dolichostenomelia (disproportionately long limbs), arachnodactyly (long thin fingers), various types of thoracic deformities, scoliosis, kyphosis and lordosis of the spine, "straight back" syndrome, flat feet, etc. These changes are associated with disruption of cartilage structure and delayed maturation of the epiphyseal growth zone, which is manifested by elongation of tubular bones. Inferiority of rib cartilages is the basis of thoracic deformities.

• Changes in the skin: hyperelasticity, thinning, tendency to traumatization and formation of keloid scars or "tissue paper" scars.

• Changes in the muscular system: decrease in muscle mass, including cardiac and oculomotor muscles, resulting in decreased myocardial contractility and myopia.

• Joint pathology: excessive mobility (hypermobility), tendency to dislocations and subluxations due to weakness of the ligamentous apparatus.

• Visual pathology: one of the most frequent manifestations of DST is represented by various degrees of myopia, lens dislocation, increased eyeball length, flat cornea, blue sclera syndrome.

• Lesions of the cardiovascular system are very diverse and often determine the prognosis. Anatomic changes of the heart valves are usually diagnosed: dilatation of fibrous rings and prolapses, abnormal chordae, dilation of the ascending aorta and pulmonary artery with subsequent formation of saccular aneurysms. In addition, thoracic and spinal deformities lead to the development of various types of thoracodiaphragmatic heart.

• Vascular damage is manifested by aneurysmal dilatations of medium and small caliber arteries and - very often - varicose veins of the lower extremities

• Bronchopulmonary lesions involve both the bronchial tree and the alveoli. Bronchiectasis, simple and cystic hypoplasia, bullous emphysema and spontaneous pneumothorax are most commonly diagnosed.[2,11,12,13,31,32,33].

There are no universal pathologic lesions of connective tissue that would form a specific phenotype. Each defect in each patient is unique in its own way. At the same time, the comprehensive distribution of connective tissue in the body determines the multiorgan nature of lesions in connective tissue dysplasia. In this regard, a classification approach with the isolation of syndromes associated with dysplastic-dependent changes and pathologic conditions is proposed [3,4,5].

Syndrome of neurological disorders: autonomic dysfunction syndrome (vegetative dystonia, panic attacks, etc.), hemicrania. Vegetative dysfunction syndrome is formed in a significant number of patients with connective tissue dysplasia one of the very first. The severity of clinical manifestations of the syndrome increases in parallel with the severity of connective tissue dysplasia. Autonomic dysfunction is observed in 97% of hereditary syndromes, and in undifferentiated connective tissue dysplasia in 78% of patients [9,10,11].

Asthenic syndrome: decreased performance, impaired tolerance of physical and psychoemotional loads, increased fatigue. Asthenic syndrome is detected in preschool and especially bright in school, adolescence and young age, accompanying patients with connective tissue dysplasia throughout life. There is a dependence of the severity of clinical manifestations of asthenia on the age of patients: the older the patients, the more subjective complaints [10,26,27].

Valve syndrome: isolated and combined prolapses of heart valves, myxomatous degeneration of valves. The valve syndrome begins to form also in childhood (4-5 years of age). Auscultatory signs of mitral valve prolapse are detected at different ages: from 4 to 34 years, but most often at the age of 12-14 years. It should be noted that echocardiographic data are in a dynamic state: more pronounced changes are noted at follow-up examinations, which reflects the influence of age on the state of the valve apparatus. In addition, the severity of valve changes is influenced by the severity of connective tissue dysplasia and ventricular volume [10,11,18].

Thoracodiaphragmatic syndrome: asthenic chest shape, chest deformities (funnel-shaped, keel-shaped), spinal deformities (scoliosis, kyphoscoliosis, hyperkyphosis, hyperlordosis, etc.), changes in diaphragm standing and excursion [3,4]. Among patients with connective tissue dysplasia, funnel-shaped thoracic deformity is the most common, keel-shaped deformity is the second most common, and asthenic thoracic shape is the most rarely detected. The beginning of the formation of thoracodiaphragmatic syndrome falls on the early school age, the distinctness of manifestations falls on the age of 10-12 years, the maximum expression of the period of 14-15 years. In all cases, funnel-shaped deformity is noted by doctors and parents 2-3 years earlier than keel-shaped deformity. The presence of thoracodiaphragmatic syndrome determines a decrease in the respiratory surface of the lungs, deformation of the lumen of the trachea and bronchi; displacement and rotation of the heart, "twisting" of the main vascular trunks. Qualitative (variant of deformation) and quantitative (degree of deformation) characteristics of thoracodiaphragmatic syndrome determine the nature and severity of changes in morphofunctional parameters of the heart and lungs. Deformations of the sternum, ribs, spine and the associated high standing of the diaphragm lead to a reduction in the thoracic cavity, increased intrathoracic pressure, disrupt blood inflow and outflow, contribute to the occurrence of cardiac arrhythmias. The presence of thoracodiaphragmatic syndrome may result in increased pressure in the small circle circulation [5,6,7,17,18].

Vascular syndrome: 1) lesions of elastic type arteries: idiopathic dilatation of the wall with formation of saccular aneurysms; 2) lesions of muscular and mixed type arteries: bifurcation-hemodynamic aneurysms, dolichoectasias of elongated and localized arterial dilatations, pathological tortuosity up to loop formation; 3)vein affection (pathological tortuosity, varicose veins of upper and lower extremities, hemorrhoidal and other. veins); 4)telangiectasia; 5)endothelial dysfunction [25,26,27,28]. Vascular changes are accompanied by increased tone in the system of large, small arteries and arterioles, decreased volume and filling rate of the arterial bed, decreased venous tone and excessive blood deposition in peripheral veins. The vascular syndrome usually manifests in adolescence and young adulthood, progressing with increasing age of patients [3,5,26,27].

Arrhythmic syndrome: ventricular extrasystole of various gradations; multifocal, monomorphic, less often polymorphic, monofocal atrial extrasystole; paroxysmal tachyarrhythmias; pacemaker migration; atrioventricular and intraventricular block; abnormalities of impulse conduction through additional pathways; ventricular preexcitation syndrome; Q-T interval prolongation syndrome. The incidence of arrhythmic syndrome is about 64% [23,26,63].

Sudden death syndrome: changes in the cardiovascular system in connective tissue dysplasia that determine the pathogenesis of sudden death - valve, vascular, arrhythmic syndromes. According to observations, in all cases the cause of death is directly or indirectly related to morphofunctional changes in the heart and vessels: in some cases it is caused by gross vascular pathology, which is easy to ascertain at autopsy (ruptured aortic aneurysms, cerebral arteries, etc.), in other cases sudden death is caused by factors that are difficult to verify on the sectional table (arrhythmic death) [12,14,28].

Bronchopulmonary syndrome: tracheobronchial dyskinesia, tracheobronchomalacia, tracheobronchomegaly, ventilation disorders (obstructive, restrictive, mixed disorders), spontaneous pneumothorax. Modern authors describe bronchopulmonary disorders in connective tissue dysplasia as genetically determined disorders of lung tissue architectonics in the form of destruction of interalveolar septa and underdevelopment of elastic and muscle fibers in small bronchi and bronchioles, leading to increased extensibility and reduced elasticity of lung tissue [34,35,40].

Immunological disorders syndrome: immunodeficiency syndrome, autoimmune syndrome, allergic syndrome. The functional state of the immune system in connective tissue dysplasia is characterized by both activation of immune mechanisms that ensure the maintenance of homeostasis and their insufficiency, leading to impaired ability to adequately release the body from foreign particles and, consequently, to the development of recurrent infectious and inflammatory diseases of the bronchopulmonary system [23,25,30].

Visceral syndrome: nephroptosis and renal dystopias, ptosis of the gastrointestinal tract, pelvic organs, dyskinesia of the gastrointestinal tract, duodenogastric and gastroesophageal refluxes, sphincter failure, esophageal diverticula, hernia of the esophageal opening of the diaphragm; ptosis of the genitals in women [23,28,30,31].

Visual pathology syndrome: myopia, astigmatism, hypermetropia, strabismus, nystagmus, retinal detachment, lens dislocation and subluxation. Accommodation disorders manifest themselves in different periods of life, in the majority of the examined patients - in school years (8-15 years) and progresses up to 20-25 years [20,21,34,35].

Hemorrhagic hematomesenchymal dysplasias: Hemoglobinopathies, Randu-Osler-Weber syndrome, recurrent hemorrhagic (hereditary platelet dysfunction, Willebrand syndrome, combined variants) and thrombotic (platelet hyperaggregation, primary antiphospholipid syndrome, hyperhomocysteinemia, factor Va resistance to activated protein C) syndromes [21,36,62].

Foot pathology syndrome: clubfoot, flat feet (longitudinal, transverse), hollow feet. Foot pathology syndrome is one of the earliest manifestations of connective tissue failure. The most common is transverse flatfoot (transverse flatfoot), in some cases combined with outward deviation of the 1st toe (hallusvalgus) and longitudinal flatfoot with pronation of the foot (flatfoot). The presence of foot pathology syndrome further reduces the possibility of physical development of patients with connective tissue dysplasia, forms a certain stereotype of life, and aggravates psychosocial problems [23,24,31].

Joint hypermobility syndrome: joint instability, joint dislocations and subluxations. The incidence of joint hypermobility is significantly higher in patients with severe connective tissue dysplasia [34,35,36].

Vertebrogenic syndrome: juvenile osteochondrosis of the spine, instability, intervertebral herniations, vertebrobasilar insufficiency; spondylolisthesis. Developing in parallel with the development of thoracodiaphragmatic syndrome and hypermobility syndrome, vertebrogenic syndrome significantly aggravates their consequences [18,19,35].

Cosmetic syndrome: dysplastic dysmorphisms of the maxillofacial region (bite anomalies, gothic palate, pronounced facial asymmetries); O- and X-shaped deformities of the limbs; skin changes (thin translucent and easily wounded skin, increased skin extensibility, "tissue paper" suture) [20,26,27,34,35]. The cosmetic syndrome of connective tissue dysplasia is significantly aggravated by the presence of small developmental anomalies detected in the absolute majority of patients with connective tissue dysplasia. The vast majority of patients have 1-5 microanomalies (hypertelorism, hypotelorism, "wrinkled" auricles, large protruding ears, low hair growth on the forehead and neck, torticollis, diastema, abnormal tooth growth, etc.)[20,26,27,60,61].

The concept of physical development. Methods of determining and assessing physical development

According to the literature [53,54,55], physical development disorders (PD) are noted in this contingent of patients.

Human physical development (PD) is understood as a set of morphological and functional features of the organism in their interrelation. Since the rate and final limit of biological potential depends on genetic and environmental factors, the child's PD is one of the most important criteria in assessing his or her state of health. The assessment of a child's FR is based on the parameters of growth, body weight, proportions of development of individual body parts, as well as the degree of development of functional abilities of the child's organism (vital capacity of lungs, muscle strength of hands, etc.; muscular development and muscle tone, the state of posture, musculoskeletal apparatus, development of subcutaneous fat layer, tissue turgor), which depend on the differentiation and maturity of cellular elements of organs and tissues, functional abilities of the nervous system and endocrine apparatus.

The methods used to study the physical development of children include: measurement of body size and weight (anthropometry), examination and description of body features and appearance (somatoscopy), dynamometry, physical performance testing with step test or cycle ergometry. Sometimes this complex includes some physiometric indicators (vital capacity of lungs, ECG data, etc.). The greater the number of features included in the assessment of physical development, the more accurate the assessment itself will be [53,54,55,56].

When assessing physical development, it is important to evaluate not only the region of residence, but also the type of settlement (city, village). The results of anthropometric measurements of large (at least 100-150 people), homogeneous by sex, age and other characteristics population groups are used as standards. Physical development standards always have a regional character, and within regions inhabited by different ethnic groups, standards developed separately for representatives of these groups should be used [56,57,58,59,60].

During **somatoscopy**, attention is paid to posture, physique, shape of the chest, legs, feet and joint mobility, the skin condition, fat deposition, shape of the back, chest, abdomen, legs, feet, degree of musculature development, and musculoskeletal system were assessed.

The spine is examined in the sagittal and frontal planes, determine the shape of the line formed by the spinous processes of the vertebrae, pay attention to the symmetry of the shoulder blades and the level of the shoulders, the state of the waist triangle formed by the waist line and the lowered arm. The shape of the back is characterized as normal, flat, round, roundly concave, flatly concave.

Posture is assessed as correct, slouching, kyphotic, lordotic and erect. To determine posture, visual observations are made on the position of the shoulder blades, shoulder level, and head posture.

Normal posture is defined by five traits:

1 - the location of the spinous processes of the vertebrae along a plumb line descending from the occipital tubercle and running along the gluteal crease;

2 - with the shoulder pads at the same level;

3 - with both shoulder blades at the same level;

4 - equal triangles (right and left) formed by the torso and freely lowered arms;

5 - correct curves of the spine in the sagittal plane (up to 5 cm deep in the lumbar spine and up to 2 cm deep in the cervical spine).

The shape of the legs is determined in a standing position with the heels together. The leg shape is evaluated as correct, X-shaped, O-shaped.

When examining the foot of the supporting surface, attention is paid to the width of the isthmus connecting the heel area to the forefoot, as well as plantography. A distinction is made between normal, flattened and flat feet.

When examining the thorax, its shape, symmetry in breathing of both halves of the thorax and type of breathing are noted. The shape of the chest, according to constitutional types, is defined as normosthenic, asthenic, hypersthenic, mixed.

The normosthenic form of the chest is characterized by proportionality of the ratio between the anteroposterior and transverse dimensions of the chest, supra- and subclavian spaces are moderately expressed. The shoulder blades are tightly adjoined to the thorax, intercostal spaces are not sharply expressed. The supracostal angle is close to the right angle and is approximately 90°.

Asthenic thorax is rather flat because the anteroposterior dimension is reduced in relation to the transverse dimension. The supra- and subclavian spaces are depressed, and the scapulae are set back from the thorax. The edge of the X rib is free and easily identified on palpation. The supracostal angle is acute - less than 90°.

Hypersthenic shape of the thorax. Its anteroposterior diameter is greater than normosthenic, and therefore the transverse section approaches a circle. The intercostal spaces are narrow, and the supra- and subclavian spaces are poorly defined. The supracostal angle is obtuse, greater than 90°.

Pathological forms of the thorax develop under the influence of disease processes in the organs of the thoracic cavity or skeletal deformities.

The shape of the chest can also be affected by different types of spinal curvature. For example, kyphotic curvature of the spine is often combined with simultaneous scoliosis and is called kyphoscoliosis, and the thorax is kyphoscoliotic.

When examining the chest, it is also necessary to pay attention to the type of breathing, its frequency, depth and rhythm. The following types of respiration are distinguished: thoracic, abdominal and mixed. If respiratory movements are performed mainly due to the contraction of intercostal muscles, then talk about the thoracic, or rib, type of breathing. It is inherent mainly in women. Abdominal type of breathing is characteristic of men. Mixed type, in which the lower chest and upper abdomen are involved in breathing, is characteristic of athletes.

Muscle development is characterized by the amount of muscle tissue, its elasticity, relief, etc. The development of musculature is additionally judged by the position of the shoulder blades, the shape of the abdomen, etc. Muscular development largely determines the strength, endurance of a person and the type of sport he/she is engaged in.

Body build is determined by size, shape, proportion (the ratio of one body size to another) and the relationship between body parts. Body build is influenced by sport, nutrition, environment (climatic conditions) and other factors. There are different types of constitution: hypersthenic, asthenic and normosthenic.

At hyperstenic type of a physique transverse sizes of a body prevail, the head rounded form, the face wide, a neck short and thick, a thorax wide and short, the abdomen big, limbs short and thick, skin dense.

Asthenic type of physique is characterized by predominance of longitudinal dimensions of the body. Asthenics have a narrow face, long and thin neck, long and flat chest, small abdomen, thin limbs, underdeveloped muscles, thin pale skin.

The normosthenic type of physique is characterized by a proportional physique.

The dependence of a person's constitutional type and his or her susceptibility to certain diseases has been noticed. Thus, asthenics are more likely to have tuberculosis, gastrointestinal tract diseases, while hyperstenics have metabolic diseases, liver diseases, hypertension, etc.

Measurement of flexibility (mobility) of the spinal column and peripheral joints.

Flexibility is the ability to perform movements of wide amplitude. The measure of flexibility is the maximum amplitude of movements. A distinction is made between active and passive flexibility. Active flexibility is performed by the subject himself, passive - under the influence of an external force (in patients - with the help of an LFC methodologist). Flexibility depends on the condition of joints, elasticity (extensibility) of ligaments, muscles, age, ambient temperature, biorhythms, time of day, etc.

When measuring joint mobility, a bar goniometer is used, consisting of a movable bar and a gravity goniometer (in degrees). Joint mobility is measured in flexion and extension Joints have a physiologic range of motion, and forcibly increasing it is not safe for health.

In **anthropometry**, the following are measured: Standing height, sitting height, weight, paused chest circumference (PCC), inhalation PCC, exhalation PCC, lung excursion, waist circumference, shoulder circumference, forearm circumference, thigh circumference, shin circumference, shoulder diameter (D), D frontal thorax, D sagital thorax, D of pelvis, D of distal shoulder, D of distal forearm, D of distal thigh, D of distal tibia, measurement of hand muscle strength - dynamometry, measurement of back muscle strength (back strength), measurement of vital capacity of lungs (VCL) by spirometry.

The level of physical development is determined by a set of methods based on measurements of morphological and functional features. There are basic and additional anthropometric indicators. The first include height, body weight, chest circumference (at maximum inhalation, pause and maximum exhalation), hand strength and standing strength (strength of back muscles). In addition, the main indicators of physical development include determination of the ratio of "active" and "passive" body tissues (lean mass, total body fat) and other indicators of body composition. Additional anthropometric indicators include sitting height, neck circumference, abdomen, waist, thigh, shin, shoulder, sagittal and frontal diameters of the chest, arm length, and others. Thus, anthropometry includes determination of lengths, diameters, circumferences, etc.

The obtained anthropometric indices are evaluated by index and percentile methods.

Indices of physical development. These are physical development indices representing the ratio of various anthropometric traits expressed in a priori mathematical formulas.

The following indices are used to assess the physical development of patients: weight-bearing index (Kettle), Erisman index (index of proportionality of chest development), vital index, strength indices, Pinier index (index of physique strength), Pirke index (proportionality coefficient). Formulas for calculating the indices are given in Appendix 1.

The *centile method* gives a real characteristic of indicators in a condensed form. The essence of the method is that all variants of the studied trait are arranged in classes from the minimum to the maximum value and by mathematical transformation the whole series is divided into 100 parts. Columns of centile tables show the boundaries of the measured attribute for a certain percentage (or centile) of all children of the age-sex group.

A scale is used in which the boundaries of 3 (5), 10, 25, 50, 75, 90, 97(95) centiles are provided. The sizes of all centile intervals are not the same.

Two types of centile standards are most commonly used to monitor development: univariate centile scales (assessing the distribution of traits relative to sex and age) and graphs (nomograms showing the distribution of body weight relative to body length).

In mass examinations of children, one-dimensional centile tables are recommended for evaluating the main anthropometric indices, selecting groups with "borderline" values and possible pathological deviations of features. Practical use of these tables is simple and convenient. Each measured trait is placed in its corridor (interval) of the centile scale in the corresponding table. Depending on the number of the centile interval, which reflects its position in the row, an evaluation judgment is formulated and a medical decision is made in accordance with the following scheme:

The 1st centile interval is the area of "low" values, occurs rarely (not more than 3 or 5%) in healthy children, the child requires examination or counseling - "Diagnostic Group". There is one historically established peculiarity - when assessing anthropometric indicators, the 1st and 8th c.i. are usually taken as 3% and 97% cut-off points, and BMI (BMI) and hemodynamic indicators - 5% and 95% cut-off points, respectively.

2nd centile interval - from 3(5) to 10 centiles, the area of "reduced" values, occurs in 7(5)% of healthy children, the child is indicated for counseling in the presence of other health or developmental abnormalities - "Attention Group".

The *3rd centile interval* is from 10th to 25th centile, an area of "below average" values, found in 15% of healthy children;

The *4th centile interval* - from 25 to 50 centiles, the area of "average" values, occurs in 25% of healthy children.

The 50th centile represents the median;

The *5th centile interval* - from 50 to 75 centiles, the area of "medium-high" values, occurs in 25% of healthy children;

The *6th centile interval* - from 75 to 90 centiles, the area of "elevated" values, occurs in 15% of healthy children;

7th centile interval - 90 to 97(95) centiles, an area of "elevated" values, occurs in 7(5)% of healthy children, counseling is indicated in the presence of other health or developmental abnormalities - "Attention Group".

8th centile interval - from 97(95) centile, the area of "high" values, occurs rarely (not more than 3(5)%) in healthy children, there is a high probability of pathological nature of changes, the child requires examination or counseling - "Diagnostic Group".

For screening examinations, it is suggested that values in 3 to 6 centile intervals (10 to 90 centiles) found in 80% of healthy children should be considered as variants of the norm.

On the basis of centile estimations of body length (BL), body mass (BM) and chest circumference (CC) determine the harmony of the morphological state of the organism. Optimal ratios of these indicators provide perfect functioning of the musculoskeletal apparatus, cardiovascular, respiratory and other systems of the organism. The diagnosis of obesity is based on the correspondence of these indicators. If the difference in the number of centile intervals between any two of the above-mentioned indicators does not exceed 1, the development should be considered harmonious. If this difference is 2, the development is disharmonious, and if the difference is 3 intervals or more, we are talking about sharply disharmonious, or heterochronic, development.

Evaluation on a unidimensional centile scale provides a means of calculating tempo somatotype.

Temporal somatotype is a characteristic of a child's growth rate determined on the basis of DT, MT, and OGC centile numbers and reflecting the child's biological age. Somatotype is calculated as the sum of centile interval numbers (age-sex scale) for length, body weight, and chest circumference. There are 3 types of age development rates:

1   .*MICROSOMATIC type*, characterizing slowed rate of age development - sum of scores from 3 to 10.

2   .*MESOSOMATIC type* characterizing average growth rate - sum of scores from 11 to 17. This type can be divided into 2 subtypes:

a)   Micromesosomatic - a sum of 11 to 13 points, with a moderately slow growth rate;

б)   Macromesosomatic - a sum of 14 to 17 points with a moderately accelerated growth rate.

3.*MACROSOMATIC type* characterized by accelerated rates of development - sum of scores from 18 to 24.

Peculiarities of physical development in DST

On somatoscopy, the physique of many children with DST is irregular, with cosmetic syndrome in the form of various deformities of the maxillofacial area (MFA), as well as various types of posture disorders and abnormal chest shape.

Children suffering from DST also have O-shaped and X-shaped deformities of the limbs, flattened form of the foot, flat feet of I-, II- and III-degree.

Examination of the skin and visible mucous membranes reveals pallor of the skin and visible mucous membranes, icteric sclerae and bluish coloration around the eyes.

The majority of children have poor development of subcutaneous fatty tissue and muscular system, and the musculoskeletal apparatus (MSA) shows hypermobility of joints.

Children with DST often have funnel-shaped rib cage, rachitic, navicular, etc.

Chapter II. Application of physical factors in rehabilitation of children with connective tissue dysplasia

An important condition for effective rehabilitation of patients with various nosologic forms of connective tissue dysplasia (CTD) is the correct choice of medical means: non-medication, medication or surgery. Literature data [16,19,25,32,37,41,43,49] formulate the basic principles of treatment of these patients:

1.   **Non-medicamentous therapy** (adequate regimen, diet, physical therapy, massage, physio- and electrotherapy, psychotherapy, sanatorium-resort treatment, orthopedic correction, vocational guidance) [41,43].

2.   **Diet therapy** (use of foods enriched with protein, vitamins and trace elements).

3.   **Drug symptomatic therapy** (treatment of pain syndrome, improvement of venous blood flow, administration of beta-blockers, adaptogens, sedatives, hepatoprotectors, surgical treatment, etc.). [16,19].

4.   **Pathogenetic therapy** (stimulation of collagen formation, correction of disorders of synthesis and catabolism of glycosoaminoglycans, stabilization of mineral and vitamin metabolism, improvement of bioenergetic state of the organism) [32,37,41].

Basic principles of non-medication therapy

In the absence of significant functional disorders of the leading organs and systems, patients with DST are shown a general regimen with proper alternation of work (study) and rest. Exceptions are patients with osteogenesis imperfecta, who need to lead a gentle lifestyle (wear corsets, use crutches, avoid traumatization) in order to prevent fractures. Patients with osteoarthritis on the background of DST should limit the load on the affected joints. They are not recommended running, jumping, lifting and carrying weights, squatting, fast walking, especially on rough terrain, climbing uphill and walking on stairs. It is advisable to avoid fixed positions, such as prolonged sitting or standing in one position, which worsens blood flow to the diseased joints [12,16,17,25]. When the joints of the upper extremities are affected, carrying heavy weights, pushing heavy things by hand, playing musical instruments, typing on a tight keyboard should be limited. The rhythm of optimal motor activity for patients with osteoarthritis on the background of DST is a reasonable alternation of load (10-15 minutes) with periods of rest (5-10 minutes), during which the joint should be unloaded in a lying or sitting position. To restore blood circulation after loading, several joint movements (flexion, extension, cycling) should be performed in the same positions [25,32,37,41].

Therapeutic massage - relieves painful muscle spasm, improves blood supply, nerve impulse transmission, trophic muscles of the trunk and joints. Recently, a widespread use of spot massage with a beam of HeNe laser, which has a biostimulating, analgesic, sedative effect. Procedures are carried out daily or at intervals of one or two days, it is desirable to take at least three courses of treatment (15-20 sessions) with an interval of one month. Underwater massage produces favorable results [25,32,37].

Peculiarities of physiotherapy in children

The peculiarities of application of physiotherapy methods in children is conditioned by age-related anatomo-physiological differences and peculiarities of pathology. The child's body differs not only in smaller size, but also qualitatively, it is constantly growing, developing, which limits the adaptive capabilities. The disease often leads to delayed development. The task of applying physical factors are the prevention and treatment of diseases, as well as ensuring the development of all systems and functions in accordance with age. When selecting factors should take into account the age of the child, the nature, stage of the disease and the mechanism of action of the factor. Important is the choice of methods, parameters of exposure depending on individual reactivity, especially in allergic children. At the same time, methods of non-medicinal treatment are especially important in allergic diseases, allowing to reduce the dose of drugs, level their side effects.

In childhood, physical methods play an essential role in the prevention of diseases, increasing the resistance of the child's body to unfavorable external and internal influences.

Galvanization and drug electrophoresis are used in children from 2-3 weeks of life. Maximum current density for children up to 1 year of life - 0.01 - 0.02 mA/cm^2 duration - up to 10 minutes; in preschool age - 0.03-0.05 and 10-15 minutes respectively; over 7 years - from 0.05 to 0.07 mA/cm^2 and up to 1520 minutes; for a course of treatment from 10 to 12-15 procedures.

Different electrode placement is used: transverse, longitudinal, segmental-reflex, endonasal, according to Vermel.

Low-frequency magnetotherapy is a method that uses exposure to an alternating magnetic field of low frequency. This factor is well tolerated by children and has a mild analgesic effect. Dosage the effects of PMPNF on the inductance in millitesla (mTl) and time of exposure (children are used from 9.8 to 25 mTl, which corresponds to 1-4 position of the intensity indicator). Duration of the procedures carried out daily, from 10-15 to 20 minutes; for the course of treatment from 10 -15 minutes to 20 procedures.

Ultrasound in pediatric practice is used with a frequency of 880 and 2640 kHz; these frequencies provide penetration of vibrations respectively to a depth of 4-5 or 1.5 - 2 cm. 2640 mHz frequency is recommended in the treatment of skin focal inflammatory diseases. Ultrasound for children is not used on the growth zones of bones. In drug phonophoresis for children older than 3-5 years use pulse mode and intensity from 0.1 to 0.3 W/cm^2 , children under 3 years of age ultrasound therapy is carried out only for special indications at an intensity of 0.05 to 0.1 to 0.3-W/cm2 (for older schoolchildren with contractures). Duration of exposure from 2-3 to 5 minutes per field, for a course of treatment from 6-8 to 10 procedures conducted every other day.

In physiotherapy of sick children, it is necessary to take into account, in addition to age, the peculiarities of reactivity: allergic mood of the organism may cause an inadequate response. Children with neurotic reactions require more attention. The child can not always correctly assess their feelings, so it is important to observe his behavior, facial expressions, skin coloration. The effectiveness of treatment depends largely on the behavior of the staff: a calm environment, friendly contact with the child, confidence in success improve the results. It is important not to overload the child with procedures.

General contraindications to the use of physical factors are: severe general condition, febrile body temperature, active tuberculosis, increased bleeding, circulatory failure, kidney function, liver function, severe hypotrophy, malignant neoplasms. There are contraindications to the use of certain factors: photosensitization - for UV radiation, violation of thermosensitivity - for thermal procedures, the presence of epileptic syndrome - for electrostimulation and other electrical procedures, drug allergy - for the use of this drug by aerosols, electrophoresis.

Features of electrode application to children:

1.   the current strength (or density) is less:

-     up to 1 year - 0.01 mA/cm^2

- 1 to 2 years - 0.02 mA/cm^2

- 3 to 5 years - 0.03 mA/cm^2

- from 6 to 10 years - 0.04 mA/cm^2

- from 11 to 14 years of age - 0.05 mA/cm^2

- 15 to 17 years of age - 0.06 mA/cm^2

2. electrodes small from 50 cm^2 to 150 cm^2

3. pocket pads

4. and tie it off with rubberized elastic bandages.

5. fixation of the electrode with a bag filled with sand

6. the device is kept out of the reach of children

7. current-carrying wires must be soldered to lead electrodes

8. The shield on the plating board shall be turned on at 5 milliamperes.

Application of physical factors in preoperative and early postoperative periods

A mandatory step in the management of DST patients after a comprehensive examination and diagnosis is a competent discussion between the doctor and the patient before starting rehabilitation therapy. It is necessary to gain the confidence of both the patient and his parents in the possibility of a reliable improvement in the quality of life and restoration of lost adaptive skills.

Physiotherapeutic treatment is used according to the indications. Thus, in imperfect osteogenesis to accelerate fracture healing, in osteoporosis of various genesis recommended electrophoresis of 5% calcium chloride solution, 4% magnesium sulfate solution, 2% copper sulfate solution or 2% zinc sulfate solution on the collar zone or locally. In the syndrome of vegetovascular dystonia vagotonic type, often concomitant DST, apply 1% solution of caffeine sodium-benzoate, ephedrine hydrochloride or mesaton - on the collar method or the method of ion reflexes according to Shcherbak. To stimulate the function of the adrenal cortex, drug electrophoresis with 1.5% etomizole and DMV on the adrenal area is used. To normalize vascular tone prescribe water procedures that provide "gymnastics" vessels: general carbon dioxide, coniferous, hydrochloride, hydrogen sulfide and radon baths. At home are available dousing, rubbing, contrast shower, salt-coniferous and foam baths. A very useful physiotherapeutic method of treatment - sauna (air temperature - 100 ° C, relative humidity - 10-12%, duration of stay - 30 minutes), the course - 25 sessions for 3-4 months. Magneto-, inducto- and laser therapy, electrophoresis with Dimexide (dimethyl sulfoxide) are widely used to improve cartilage nutrition.

In order to soften dense connective tissue formations (e.g., postoperative keloid scars), DST patients undergo phonophoresis. Collalysin (collagenase), 0.2% solution of hydrocortisone, water-soluble succinate, lidase, fibrinolysin are used for this purpose. Electrophoresis according to the 4-electrode technique of ascorbic acid, sulfur, zinc, copper; chromotherapy (green, red matrix) according to the general technique are widely used [25,32,41,43,49].

Chapter III. Application of therapeutic physical training at the stages of rehabilitation

In the absence of significant functional disorders of the leading organs and systems, patients with DST are shown a general regimen with proper alternation of work (study) and rest. Exceptions are patients with osteogenesis imperfecta, who need to lead a gentle lifestyle (wear corsets, use crutches, avoid traumatization) in order to prevent fractures. Patients with osteoarthritis on the background of DST should limit the load on the affected joints. They are not recommended running, jumping, lifting and carrying weights, squatting, fast walking, especially on rough terrain, climbing uphill and walking on stairs. It is advisable to avoid fixed positions, such as prolonged sitting or standing in one position, which worsens blood flow to the diseased joints. When the joints of the upper extremities are affected, it is necessary to limit the carrying of heavy weights, pushing heavy things by hand, playing musical instruments, typing on a tight keyboard. The rhythm of optimal motor activity for patients with osteoarthritis on the background of DST is a reasonable alternation of load (10-15 minutes) with periods of rest (5-10 minutes), during which the joint should be unloaded in a lying or sitting position. To restore blood circulation after loading, several joint movements (flexion, extension, cycling) should be performed in the same positions.

Therapeutic physical training (TPT) is a method of natural biological content, which is based on the use of the main biological function of the organism - movement. The function of movement is the main stimulator of the processes of growth, development and formation of the organism. The function of movement is the main stimulator of the processes of growth, development and formation of the organism. The function of movement, stimulating the active activity of all systems of the organism, supports and develops them, contributing to the increase in the overall performance of the patient.

LFC is a method of nonspecific therapy, and the applied physical exercises are nonspecific stimuli. Any physical exercise always involves all parts of the nervous system in a response.

LFK as a method of pathogenetic therapy. Systematic application of physical exercises is able to influence the reactivity of the body, to change both the general reaction of the patient and its local manifestation.

LFC is a method of active functional therapy. Regular dosed training with physical exercises stimulates, trains and adapts individual systems and the whole organism of the patient to increasing physical loads, eventually leading to functional adaptation of the patient [11,20,25].

Physical therapy is indicated for all patients with DST. Regular (3-4 times a week, 20-30 minutes) moderate physical training aimed at strengthening the muscles of the back, abdomen, and limbs is recommended. Exercises are performed in a non-contact static-dynamic mode, in the supine position. Physical exercises should not increase the load on the ligamentous-articular apparatus and increase the mobility of joints and spine. The method of physical therapy should always be discussed with a specialist. It is necessary to take into account the nature of the pathology, clinical and radiological, biochemical criteria of the lesion of the musculoskeletal system. It is useful to prescribe complexes of exercises performed in the supine or abdominal position [41,43]. Most patients are contraindicated from hanging and spinal traction, contact sports, isometric training, weightlifting, and carrying large weights. Hydroprocedures, therapeutic swimming, which relieves static load on the spine, have a good effect.

Aerobic training of the cardiovascular system is recommended: dosed walking, skiing, traveling, hiking, jogging, comfortable cycling. Useful dosed physical activity on exercise machines and exercise bikes, badminton, table tennis, exercises with light dumbbells, breathing exercises. Systematic physical activity increases the adaptive capacity of the cardiovascular system. However, in the presence of signs of its damage - myocardiodystrophy, cardiomyopathy, myxomatous degeneration and significant valve leaflet prolapse, aortic root dilatation - excessive physical or mental exertion, participation in any sports competitions is strictly prohibited [11,12,16,17,19]. All patients with DST should not engage in professional sports and dancing, as excessive loads on functionally inferior connective tissue will lead to extremely rapid onset of its decompensation [43].

Results of own research

126 patients aged from 5 to 17 years with the diagnosis of TMDT with the leading cosmetic syndrome accompanied by various deformities of the BFD, confirmed clinically and instrumentally, were examined. There were 53 (42%) boys and 73 (68%) girls who were distributed by age groups (Table 1).

Table 1.

Distribution of patients by age groups

Paul	Age, years												
	5-6		7	8	9	10	11	12	13	14	15	16	17
Mal, n	4	10	8	4	2	8	6	2	4	1	-	3	2
Dev, n	2	5	10	2	8	7	1	6	6	10	8	5	3

The physical development of children was studied by somatoscopy and anthropometry methods.

Clinical and functional characteristics of patients and assessment of physical development

At somatoscopy, the following results were obtained:

The physique was assessed as "correct" in 47% and "incorrect" in 53% of children.

У 100% of the examined children had cosmetic syndrome in the form of various deformities of the maxillofacial region (MFR).

У 87% of children had various types of posture disorders and 43% had abnormal chest shape (Table 4).

Correct leg shape was noted in 36% of children, 41% had O-shaped and 23% had X-shaped limb deformities.

The correct foot shape was observed in 17%, flattened - in 35%, flat feet of I-degree - in 29%, II-degree - in 16% and III-degree - in 3% of children.

When assessing the condition of the skin and visible mucous membranes it was noted: clear and normal color - in 58%, pallor of the skin and visible mucous membranes - in 27%, ichtericity of the sclera - in 5% and bluish coloration around the eyes - in 5% of the examined.

У weak subcutaneous fatty tissue development was observed in the majority of the examined subjects.

When studying the state of the muscular system, it was revealed that - 12% of children have a moderately developed muscular system, 82% have a poorly developed muscular system, and no good development was noted.

In the examination of the musculoskeletal system (MS), joint hypermobility was detected in 17% of subjects.

Anthropometric indices were studied within age groups: 6, 7, 8, 8, 9, 10, 11, 12, 12, 13, 14, 15, 16, 17 years old. The obtained results are reflected in Table 2.

Table 2.

The main anthropometric indices of different age groups.

Age groups.	Indicators				
	Standing height	Body weight	OKG in pause	Exh. GC	GI
5 years	102,43±1,08	16,25±0,47	52,37±0,77	3,81±0,21	618,75±39,37
6 years old	112,28±0,92	17,5±0,47	54,14±0,48	4,14±0,29	778,5±40,77
7 years	1,23±1,23	0,48±0,48	0,68±0,68	0,33±0,33	37,83±37,83
8 years	2,11±2,1	0,56±0,56	0,53±0,53	0,27±0,27	57,42±57,42
9 years old	125,60±1,23	20,65±0,28	58,90±0,85	4,8±0,21	1080±65,39
10 years	138,30±1,98	28,09±0,84	63,53±0,80	5,15±0,24	1146,1±59,02
11 years old	139,66±1,36	29,5±1,36	66,42±0,35	6,1±0,18	1485,71±49,62
12 years	147±0,70	32,5±0,93	66,08±0,68	5,58±0,29	1766,66±0,22
13 years old	150,25±1,87	36,37±1,34	68,8±0,78	6,3±0,42	1485±104,13
14 years old	158±0,79	42,78±1,51	82,07±1,17	4,78±0,18	34,42±80,7
15 years	152,5±1,60	38,41±0,80	77,56±1,35	5,1 ±0,24	1257,28±56,55
16 years old	162,18±1,40	44,33±0,70	78,18±0,83	6,62±0,32	1362,5±76,84
17 years old	159,2±2,22	53,5±0,46	80,8±0,84	4,4±0,28	2220±173,9

Anthropometric indices were evaluated using the index and centile method.

Assessment of the index method showed that at the age of 6-9 years a decrease in body mass index (BMI) was found in 34%, in 10-13 years - in 67% and in 14-17 years - in 92% of the examined. Decrease in mass growth index (MGI) at the age of 6-10 years was detected in 28.5% of children and at the age of 11-17 years - in 91.6%. Weak indices reflecting the function of the respiratory system were noted. The Erisman index, which characterizes the proportionality of chest development, was reduced in 79% of 6-7 year olds and in 83.6% of 8-17 year olds; reduction of the vital index in 6-10 year olds in 23% and in 11-17 year olds in 63%. Force dynamometry indices confirmed the data of somatoscopy: in all age groups, 86.5% of children in all age groups had significantly lower than normal hand muscle strength and static strength.

Three main indicators (height, body weight and chest circumference at pause) were analyzed using the centile method (Table 3). Centile evaluation showed that 55% of children were classified in the I, II and III intervals (zone of reduced and low values) for height, 76% and 53% for body weight and chest circumference, respectively.

In determining the tempo somatotype, microsomatic type was found in- 55% of children, mesosomatic type in- 45% of children.

In general, the physical development of children was assessed as disharmonious and sharply disharmonious. In the comparative assessment of physical development by age groups, a high percentage of disharmoniously and sharply disharmoniously developed children with increasing indicators in older age groups was determined.

Table 3: Table of results of physical development assessment of children with connective tissue dysplasia using the centile method (%)

Age	n	Mesosomatic type	Microsomatic type	Macrosomatic type	Harmonic.	Dis-harmonious.	Dramatically disharmonious.	Body weight deficiency	Normal body weight	Overweight	Normal growth	Low stature
7 years	18	11	67	11	28	17	55	56	33	11	85	15
8 years	4	10	90	0	0	50	50	75	25	0	75	25
9 years old	10	30	70	0	0	10	90	60	40	0	80	20
10 years	15	47	53	0	0	40	60	60	40	0	53	47
11 years old	7	43	57	0	14	29	57	71	29	29	100	0
12 years	8	13	87	0	25	13	62	63	37	0	86	14
13 years	10	20	50	30	20	20	60	60	30	10	83	0

old												
14 years old	11	45	45	10	9	27	64	64	36	0	86	14
15 years	8	34	66	0	0	2	88	88	12	0	83	0
16 years old	8	37	63	0	13	13	74	88	12	0	86	14
17 years old	5	20	80	0	0	20	80	71	29	0	85	15
total	104	31	63	6	12	20	68	65	33	2	87	13

Evaluation of the Stange and Henchy breath tests revealed baseline low inspiratory and expiratory breath-hold scores.

Thus, the obtained data indicate the presence of a pronounced delay in physical development in children with dysplastic syndrome and progression in older age groups.

From the results obtained, it can be concluded that it is necessary to apply special rehabilitation programs with the use of dosed physical loads.

Methods of physical development correction, application of physical therapy complexes

In the rehabilitation of children with DST, the method of physical therapy was used with the application of a developed special set of exercises for children with DST. An example set of exercises is presented in Appendix 2.

The examined children were randomly divided into two groups depending on the rehabilitation program:

- in the first group (main group) therapeutic gymnastics procedures were performed;

- children of the second group (control group) did not undergo LFC.

The main goals of LFC in this contingent were:

- improvement of psycho-physiological status of patients;

- normalization of the correlative function of the CNS;

- Strengthening of all muscle groups;

- strengthening back muscles and correcting posture;

- improved external respiration;

- increase in vital capacity;

- improving the trophicity of the facial tissue of the affected area;

- improving the condition of the masticatory muscles;

- restoration of impaired mouth opening and chewing function.

Therapeutic gymnastics procedures were performed in the morning for 20-30 minutes, daily, using individual or small-group methods, for a course of 10-15 procedures. The reaction to the load was evaluated clinically (presence of complaints, skin color, sweating level, child's reaction to the instructor's commands) and by HR. At the end of the course of treatment, children and their parents were given detailed instructions and recommendations on how to continue the exercise program at their place of residence.

The repeated course of treatment was carried out after 4-6 months. The dynamics of the children's condition was evaluated every 6 months.

The criteria of the effectiveness of the rehabilitation measures were the dynamics of GI, GI, OHC in pause, chest excursion, and Stange and Henchey tests characterizing the functional state of the respiratory system, as well as the amplitude of movements in the temporomandibular joint and the severity of pain syndrome in the postoperative zone in children who underwent reconstructive surgeries on the maxillofacial region.

Stange test (breath holding on inhalation). After 5-7 min of rest in a sitting position, the subject took a full inhalation and exhalation, and then inhaled again (80-90% of the maximum) closing the mouth and nose. The time from the moment of delay to its cessation was noted. The duration of breath-holding depends to a great extent on the volitional efforts of a person, therefore, in breath-holding there is a distinction between the time of pure breath-holding and the volitional component. The beginning of the latter was recorded by the first contraction of the diaphragm (abdominal wall oscillation). In healthy children and adolescents aged 6-18 years, the duration of breath-hold on inhalation ranges from 16-55 seconds.

Genci's test (breath holding on exhalation). The subject, after a full exhalation and inhalation, exhales again and holds the breath.Healthy untrained persons can hold the breath on exhalation for 20-30 seconds.

Children who underwent reconstructive surgeries on the maxillofacial region also received physiotherapeutic procedures in the pre- and postoperative periods. In order to prepare tissues for surgery, the following procedures were performed: magnetotherapy, paraffin-ozokerite applications and massage of the face, neck and collar zone in the amount of 6 to 10 procedures.

In the early postoperative period on the 3-5th day UVO and low-heat doses of UHF electric field (e.p.UHF) or magnetotherapy with a course of 6-10 procedures were administered for bacteriocidal and antiexudative therapy.

In the group of children who used a special complex of therapeutic gymnastics (TG), there was a tendency of positive dynamics of posture, chest circumference, GI, GI, functional respiratory tests.

The dynamics of the listed indicators in different age groups is reflected in Tables 4, 5, 6, 7.

Table 4.

Comparative dynamics of physical development indicators of the main group of children aged 5-7 years old

Indicators	Survey periods			
	Before treatment.	I reiterate	II repetition	III repetition
GI	803,9±36,46	804,1±36,54	850,75±36,82	900,4±37,2
GI	38,7±1,57	38,9±1,74	39,3±2,12	40,65±2,54
OKG in pause	55,69±0,69	55,92±0,81	56,32±0,94	58,75±1,45
Ex.gr. cl.	4,76±0,31	4,92±0,45	5,52±0,72	6,87±0,93
Pr. Stange	15,46±0,64	15,75±0,69	15,96±0,87	18,35±1,1
Genci Pr.	11,15±0,61	11,47±0,84	11,52±0,88	13,87±0,91

Table 5.

Comparative dynamics of physical development indicators of the main group of children aged 8-9 years old

Indicators	Survey periods			
	Before treatment.	I reiterate	II repetition	III repetition
GI	1175±84,92	1188±84,96	1192±84,97	1305±89,3

GI	41,04±3,43	41,25±3,64	41,54±3,78	45,95±3,86
OKG in pause	62,75±0,88	62,84±0,9	62,87±0,92	68,89±0,95
Ex.gr. cl.	5,75±0,09	5,82±0,12	5,86±0,18	7,92±0,29
Pr. Stange	24,5±0,23	24,78±0,29	25,2±0,46	28,65±0,74
Pr. Genche	23±0,26	23,31±0,32	23,87±0,71	29,04±0,87

Table 6.

Comparative dynamics of physical development indicators of the main group of children aged 11 -13 years old

Indicators	Survey periods			
	Before treatment.	I reiterate	II repetition	III repetition
GI	1562,5±119,2	1562,67±119,34	1562,84±119,67	1600,23±119,8
GI	42,89±2,91	42,91±2,96	43,41±3,0	48,86±3,28
OKG in pause	68,21±1,06	68,32±1,12	68,44±1,23	74,84±1,52
Ex.gr. cl.	5,14±0,40	5,62±0,53	5,76±0,61	7,89±0,75
Pr. Stange	20,75±0,31	20,86±0,43	20,92±0,57	24,2±0,71
Pr. Genche	18,75±0,23	18,84±0,37	18,95±0,45	21,05±0,72

Table 7.

Comparative dynamics of physical development indicators of the main group of children aged 14-17 years old

Indicators	Survey periods			
	Before treatment.	I reiterate	II repetition	III repetition
GI	1223,15±53,13	1223,3±53,24	1223,65±53,4	1800,83±53,52
GI	29,71±1,06	29,86±1,23	29,93±1,34	32,06±1,62
OKG in pause	76,38±0,92	76,43±1,03	76,54±1,15	84,61±1,3
Ex.gr. cl.	6,15±0,32	6,28±0,5	6,37±0,63	8,57±0,78

Pr. Stange	20,92±0,41	21,1±0,52	21,27±0,63	30,34±0,78
Pr. Genche	18,84±0,45	18,95±0,56	19±0,64	26,2±0,71

In the comparative analysis of the parameters of the main and control groups, a significant difference in the dynamics of the parameters in the course of treatment was noted. The indices of LEF, GI, chest excursion and breathing tests in the group of children without LH were significantly behind the similar indices of the main group. Comparative dynamics of indicators is reflected in Tables 8, 9, 10, 11.

Table 8.

Comparative indicators of the main and control group at the age of 5-7 years old

Indicators	Application of LFK complex	
	Main group	Control group
GI	900,4±37,2	804,1±36,54
GI	40,65±2,54	38,9±1,74
OKG in pause	58,75±1,45	55,92±0,81
Ex.gr. cl.	6,87±0,93	4,92±0,45
Pr. Stange	18,35±1,1	15,75±0,69
Pr. Genche	13,87±0,91	11,47±0,84

Table 9.

Comparative performance of the main and control group at the age of 8-10 years.

Indicators	Application of LFK complex	
	Main group	Control group
GI	1305±89,3	1188±84,96
GI	45,95±3,86	41,25±3,64
OKG in pause	68,89±0,95	62,84±0,9
Ex.gr. cl.	7,92±0,29	5,82±0,12
Pr. Stange	28,65±0,74	24,78±0,29

| Pr. Genche | 29,04±0,87 | 23,31±0,32 |

Table 10.

Comparative indicators of the main and control group at the age of 11-13 years old

Indicators	Application of LFK complex	
	Main group	Control group
GI	1600,23±119,8	1562,67±119,34
GI	48,86±3,28	42,91±2,96
OKG in pause	74,84±1,52	68,32±1,12
Ex.gr. cl.	7,89±0,75	5,62±0,53
Pr. Stange	24,2±0,71	20,86±0,43
Pr. Genche	21,05±0,72	18,84±0,37

Table 11.

Comparative indicators of the main and control group at the age of 14-17 years old

Indicators	Application of LFK complex	
	Main group	Control group
GI	1800,83±53,52	1223,3±53,24
GI	32,06±1,62	29,86±1,23
OKG in pause	84,61±1,3	76,43±1,03
Ex.gr. cl.	8,57±0,78	6,28±0,5
Pr. Stange	30,34±0,78	21,1±0,52
Pr. Genche	26,2±0,71	18,95±0,56

1. In children with congenital dysplasia of the maxillofacial region, somatoscopy reveals numerous abnormalities of posture, chest shape, legs and feet. Anthropometry in children with congenital dysplasia of the maxillofacial region reveals a significant decrease in physical development indicators compared to age norms. The degree of lag in physical development increases with increasing age of children. The lag of this contingent of patients in physical

development requires inclusion of special programs of dosed loads in the complex of restorative treatment. The use of regular physical training in children with dysplasia of the BFD contributes to a reliable increase in GEF, GI and breathing tests.

REFERENCE LIST

1. Anokhina VV, Bugrimov DY, Muravitskaya MN Features of the course of acute respiratory viral diseases in children with phenotypic signs of undifferentiated connective tissue dysplasia // Bulletin of New Medical Technologies. - 2011. - T. 18, № 2. - C. 224 - 227.

2. Antropova M.V. et al. Problems of children's health and physical development / M.V. Antropova, G.V. Borodkina, L.M. Kuznetsova et al. //Health of the Russian Federation. - 1999. - № 5. - C. 17-21.

3. Arsentyev V.G. et al. Connective tissue dysplasias - constitutional basis of multi-organ disorders in children and adolescents / V.G. Arsentyev, Yu. Tikhonov et al. //Pediatrics. - 2011. - T. 90, № 5.- C. 54 - 57.

4. Arsentiev VG, Staroverov YI, ShabalovN. P. Features echo structure of the heart and kidneys in connective tissue dysplasia in children // Nephrology. - 2011. - T. 15, № 4. - C. 99 - 99.

5. Bodrikova S.V. Physical development of high school students with vegetative dystonia syndrome and small anomalies of heart development // Bulletin of the East-Siberian Scientific Center SB RAMS. - 2007. -№ 3. - C. 66 - 67.

6. Budanova MV, Aslanova PA, Budanov PV Clinical manifestations and effects of correction of magnesium deficiency in children //Trudny Patient. - 2009. - № 1-2. - C. 50 - 54.

7. Vasilieva I.G. et al. Connective tissue dysplasias in urologic pathology in children / I.G. Vasilieva, V.V. Chemodanov, A.I. Strelnikov, P.V. Alexeev //Russian Pediatric Journal. Chemodanov, A.I. Strelnikov, P.V. Alekseev // Russian Pediatric Journal. - 2010. - № 5. - C. 30 - 33.

8. Vershinina M.V. Pathology of respiratory organs in connective tissue dysplasia (literature review) // **Ural** Medical Journal. - 2011. -№ 01-79. - C. 15 -21.

9. Genova O.A. et al. The state of the reproductive system in adolescents with markers of undifferentiated connective tissue dysplasia /O.A. Genova. Genova, E.V. Rakitskaya, R.V. Uchakina, V.K. Kozlov //Dalnevostochny Medical Journal. - 2010. - № 4. - C 55 - 59.

10. Glotov AV, Goltyapin VV, Lobachev AI Identification of socio-residential factors

affecting the development of connective tissue dysplasia of adolescents by the method of major factors //Fundamental Research. -2011. - № 8-2. - C. 338 - 341.

11.   Domnitskaya T.M. et al. Clinical significance of magnesium orotate use in adolescents with connective tissue dysplasia syndrome of the heart / T.M. Domnitskaya, A.V. Dyachenko, O.O. Kupriyanova, M.V. Domnitsky //Cardiology. - 2005. - T. 45, № 3. - C. 76 - 81.

12.   Dotsenko N.Y. et al. Connective tissue dysplasias in cardiology: proven and unknown /N.Ya.Dotsenko, L.V. Gerasimenko, S.S. Boev et al. //Zdravookhranenie Chuvashii. - 2011. - № 3. - C. 77 -81.

13.   Drobysheva O.V., BotvinievO.V.Functional state of cardiac and pyloric sphincters, sphincter of Oddi in children with undifferentiated connective tissue dysplasia and in the absence of dysplasia //Ros.zhurnal gastroenterologii, gepatologii, kolonoproktologii. - 2009. -№ 4. - C. 39 - 43.

14.   Evtushenko S.K., Lisovsky E.V., Evtushenko O.S. Dysplasia of connective tissue in neurology and pediatrics. - Donetsk: Izdat. dom "Zaslavsky", 2009. - 361 c.

15.   ZemtsovskyE.V.Dysplastic syndromes and phenotypes.Dysplastic heart. - SPb. OLGA, 2007. - 80 c.

16.   Ivanova E.A. et al. Prevention of health losses in adolescents with phenotypic manifestations of connective tissue dysplasia / E.A. Ivanova, O.V. Plotnikova, A.V. Glotov, V.G. Demchenko // Kazan Medical Journal. - 2012. - T. 93, № 1. - C. 93 - 97.

17.   Kadurina T.I. Hereditary collagenopathies (clinic, diagnosis, treatment, dispensary). - SPb. Nevsky Prospect, 2000. - 271 c.

18.   Kadurina T.I., Abbakumova L.N. Evaluation of the severity of undifferentiated connective tissue dysplasia in children // Medical Bulletin of the North Caucasus. - 2008. - № 2. - C. 15 - 20.

19.   Kadurina T.I., Gorbunova V.N. Modern concepts of connective tissue dysplasia // Kazan Medical Journal. - 2007. -T. 88, № 5. - C. 2 - 5.

20.   Kadurina T.I., Gorbunova V.N. Connective tissue dysplasia: Guide for doctors. - SPb. ELBI, 2009. - 714 c.

21.   Kalmykova AS, Tkacheva NV, Pavlenko MS Sexual development of adolescent girls

with connective tissue dysplasia syndrome and vegeto - vascular dysfunction // Medical Bulletin of the North Caucasus. - 2010. - T. 18, № 2. - C. 34 - 36.

22. Kerimova A.K.K., Babaev M.Sh.O., Askerova T.A.K. Population - genetic study of hereditary connective tissue dysplasia //Vestnik of Moscow State Regional University. Series: Natural Sciences. - 2010. - № 4.- C. 17 - 20.

23. Klemenov A.V. Extracardiac manifestations of undifferentiated connective tissue dysplasia // Clinical Medicine. - 2003. - T. 81, № 10. - C. 4 - 7.

24. Klemenov A.V. Undifferentiated dysplasia of connective tissue. - Moscow: Informtech, 2006. - 136 c.

25. Kondusova Y.V. et al. Problems of rehabilitation of children suffering from bronchial asthma on the background of connective tissue dysplasia / Y.V. Kondusova, E.S. Grosheva, A.V. Kryuchkova, I.A. Poletaeva // Vestnik Novye Meditsinskikh Tekhnologii. - 2011. - T. 18, № 2. - C. 282 - 284.

26. Korzhov I.S. Phenotypic and visceral signs of connective tissue dysplasia in children with diseases of the upper digestive tract // Mother and Child of Kuzbass 2007. - № 1 (28). - C. 29 - 26.

27. Kupriyanov I.A. et al. Features of facial pain in connective tissue dysplasia / I.A. Kupriyanov, O.N. Kupriyanova, V.V. Petko, A.M. Stamm // Vestnik of New Medical Technologies. - 2011. - T. 18, № 3. - C. 72 - 75.

28. Magomedova Sh.M. et al. Mitral valve prolapse in children with connective tissue dysplasia / Sh.M. Magomedova, K.A. Masuev, Y.M. Belozerov, I.M. Osmanov // Russian Herald of Perinatology and Pediatrics. - 2011. - T. 56, № 3. - C. 32 - 39.

29. Madyakin P.V. Influence of undifferentiated connective tissue dysplasia on the health of children and adolescents engaged in ballet and rhythmic gymnastics //Vrach-aspirant. - 2011. - T. 44, № 1.3. - C. 424 - 432.

30. Makolkin V.I. et al. Polymorphism of clinical manifestations of connective tissue dysplasia syndrome / V.I. Makolkin, V.I. Podzolkov, A.V. Rodionov et al. //Therapeutic Archive. - 2004. - T. 76, № 11. - C :77 - 80.

31. Mambetova A.M., Zhetishev R.A., Shabalova N.N. Expression of undifferentiated forms of connective tissue dysplasia in children with vesicoureteral reflux and reflux

nephropathy //Voprosy practical pediatrics. - 2011. - T. 6, № 3. - C. 64 - 68.

32. Martynov AI, Stepura OV, Ostroumova OD Congenital dysplasias of connective tissue // Vestnik RAMN. - 1998. - №2. - C.47 - 54.

33. Nechaeva G.I., Viktorova I.A., Druk I.V. Connective tissue dysplasia: prevalence, phenotypic signs, associations with other diseases //Vratsch. - 2006. - T. 9, № 1. - C. 19 - 23.

34. Nechaeva G.I. et al. Connective tissue dysplasia: the main clinical syndromes, formulation of diagnosis, treatment / G.I. Nechaeva, V.I. Yakovleva, V.P. Konev et al. //Lechachal Doctor. - 2008. -№ 2. - C 22 - 28.

35. Nechaikina SA, Malmberg SA Polymorphism of neurologic syndromes in connective tissue dysplasia in children and approaches to therapy // Neurological Journal. - 2011. - T. 16, № 5. - C. 19 - 23.

36. Nikolaev K.Yu., Oteva E.A., Nikolaeva A.A. Connective tissue dysplasia and multi-organ pathology of school-age children // Pediatrics. - 2006. - № 2. - C. 89 - 93.

37. Obrubov S.A., Demidova M.Y. Undifferentiated dysplasia of connective tissue: current state of the problem. Ros.ped. ophthalmologia. 2009; 4: 50-53.

38. Osipenko M.F., Skalinskaya M.I., Bitkhaeva M.V. Functional diseases of the biliary tract and syndrome of undifferentiated connective tissue dysplasia // Siberian Medical Journal (Irkutsk). - 2011. - T. 106, № 7. - C. 44 - 46.

39. Raspopova E.A. et al. Spondylolisthesis in children against the background of connective tissue dysplasia / E.A. Raspopova, A.A. Dudareva, A.I. Metalnikov, J.N. Radimova // Bulletin of the East Siberian Scientific Center SB RAMS. - 2011. - № S4. - C. 89 - 90.

40. Rumyantseva G.N. et al. Connective tissue dysplasia syndrome in boys with diseases of the reproductive system / G.N. Rumyantseva, V.N. Kartashev, T.A. Fedotova et al. //Children's Surgery. - 2011. - № 1. - C. 20 - 23.

41. Rychkova T.I. Physiological role of magnesium and the significance of its deficiency in connective tissue dysplasia in children // Pediatrics.- 2011. - T. 90, № 2. - C. 114 - 120.

42. Serov V.V., Sheher A.B. Connective tissue (functional morphology and general pathology). 2nd ed. M.: Medicine, 1981. - 312 c.

43.   Sidorov G.A. et al. Improvement of dispensary observation of children with various degrees of connective tissue dysplasia / G.A. Sidorov, A.F. Vinogradov, E.M. Kornyusho et al. //Vestnik novykh meditsinskikh tekhnologii. - 2010. - T. 17, № 4. - C. 136 - 139.

44.   Simonenko V.B. et al. Connective tissue dysplasias (hereditary collagenopathies) / V.B. Simonenko, P.A. Dulin, D.N. Panfilov et al. //Clinical Medicine. - 2006. - T. 84, № 6. - C. 62 - 68.

45.   Sichinava IV, Shishov AY, Belousova NA Features of manifestations of gastroduodenal pathology in children with connective tissue dysplasia // Pediatrics. - 2012. - T. 91, № 4. - C. 6 - 10.

46.   Streltsova EV, Kalmykova AS Family analysis of phenotypic features of connective tissue dysplasia syndrome // Medical Bulletin of the North Caucasus. - 2011. - № 1. - C. 36 - 39.

47.   Tarasova A.A. Dysplasia of connective tissue of the heart and thyroid diseases in children // Ultrasound and functional diagnostics. - 2006. - № 4. - C. 42 - 54.

48.   Torshin YI, Gromova OA. Connective tissue dysplasia, cell biology and molecular mechanisms of magnesium exposure // Russian Medical Journal. - 2008. - № 4. - C. 230 - 238.

49.   Churilina A.V. et al. The role of magnesium in connective tissue dysplasia (literature review) / A.V. Churilina, O.N. Moskalyuk, L.F. Chalaya et al. //Voprosy sovremennoi pediatria. - 2009. - № 4 (26). - C. 44 - 46.

50.   Filipenko P.S., Malooka Yu.S. Role of connective tissue dysplasia in the formation of mitral valve prolapse // Clinical Medicine. - 2006. - T. 84, № 12. - C. 13 - 19.

51.   Shabalov N.P., Arsentiev V.G. Hereditary diseases of connective tissue //Pediatrics: national guide. - Moscow: GEOTAR-Media, 2009. - T. 1. - C. 298 - 320.

52.   Yakovlev MV, Glotov AV, Nechaeva GI et al. Clinicoimmunologic analysis of clinical variants of connective tissue dysplasias //Therapeutic Archive. - 1994. - T. 66, № 5. - C. 9 - 13. Mazurin A.V. Propedeutics of pediatric diseases. Textbook for students of medical universities / A. V. Mazurin, I. M. Vorontsov. SPb: Foliant, 2001. 926 c.

53.   Yuriev V.V., Simakhodsky A.S., Voronovich N.N., Homich M.M. Growth and development of the child: for students of medical universities and pediatricians. Ed. 3e. SPb.:

Peter, 2007. 260 c.

54. Veltischev Y.E. Objective indicators of normal development and health of the child (norms of childhood). M., 2002. - 163 c.

55. Yuryev V.V., Yuryev VK, Simakhodskiy A.S. Automated system of professional examinations of the child population (system for assessing the health of the child population): method. recommendations. Л., 1991. 30 c.

56. Yampolskaya Y.A. Regional diversity and standardized assessment of physical development of children and adolescents. Pediatrics 2005; 6: 73-77.

57. Baranov A.A., Shcheplyagina L.A. Fundamental and applied research on the problems of growth and development of children and adolescents. Ross.pediatricheskiy zhurnal 2000; 5: 5-7.

58. Vorontsov I.M., Mataligina O.A.. To the problem of formation of standardized risk assessment scales in the ecology of childhood. Ecology of childhood: social and medical problems. SPb, 1994. C. 13-14.

59. Kamilova R.T., Niyazova G.T. Individual assessment of physical development of urban schoolchildren by the centile method. Educational and methodical manual. Ташкент-2007г.C.11-15.

60. Kamilova R.T., Niyazova G.T. Individual assessment of physical development of urban schoolchildren by the method of regression scales. Educational and methodical manual. Tashkent, 2007. C. 8-29

61. Behar J. et al. Corazziari E., Guelrud M., Functional Gallbladder and Sphincter of Oddi Disorders / J. Behar, E. Corazziari, M. Guelrud et al. Behar, E. Corazziari, M. Guelrud et al. //Gastroenterology. - 2006. -№ 130. -P. 1498 - 1509.

62. Bonow, R.O. et al. Guidelines for the management of patients with valvular heart disease /R.O. Bonow et al.]/Circulation. - 2006. - № 1 (8). - P. 148

63. Boudoudoudas H. Etiology of Valvular Heart Disease in the 21st century //Hellenic J. Cardiol. Cardiol. - 2002. -N 43. -P. 183 - 188.

64. Gazit Y. et al. Dysautonomia in the joint hypermobility syndrome /Y. Gazit, M/ Nahir, R. Grahame, G. Jacob //J. Am. Med. - 2003. - Vol. 15. - P. 33 - 40.

65.   Grau J.B. et al. The genetics of mitral valve prolapse /J.B.. Grau, L. Pirelli, P.J. Yuet al. //Clin. Genet.- 2007. - Vol. 72, № 4. -P. 288 - 295.

66.   Levine R.A., Slaugenhaupt S.A. Molecular genetics of mitral valve prolapse //Curr. Opin. Cardiol.- 2007. - Vol. 22, № 3. -P. 171 - 175.

67.   Malfait F. et al. The genetic basis of the joint hypermobility syndromes /Malfait F. et al. //Rheumatology. - 2006. - 45. - P. 502 -507.

68.   McRusick, V.A. Mendeli an inheritance in man: a catalog of human genes and genetic disorders .- http://www.ncbi. nlm. nih.gov /OMIM/. nih.gov /OMIM/.

69.   Romanelli P. et al. Clinical significance of cutaneous proteoglycan (mucin) infiltration in patients with mitral valve prolapse / P. Romanelli, R. Romanelli, F. Rongioletti et al. //J. Am. Am. Acad. Dermatol. - 2008. - Vol. 59, № 1. -P. 168-169.

70.   Yosefy C, Ben Barak A. Floppy mitral valve/mitral valve prolapse and genetics //J. Heart Valve Dis. Heart Valve Dis. - 2007. - Vol. 16, № 6. - P. 590 - 595.

APPENDIX

Appendix No. 1

Basic anthropometric indices (indicators) of child physical development

	Indicators	**Formula (method of calculation)**	**Index value**
1	Kettle, E K	Body mass in kg:(body length in m)2 x 100	Children have a wide range, adults have a range of 24-27
2	Massorostovoy, MPI	(Ratio of actual weight to the 5th percentile value of this indicator for a given age): (Ratio of actual body length to the 5th percentile value of this indicator for a given age) x 100	89 and below - high growth with body weight deficit 100-119 - overweight 120 and above - obesity
3	Erisman	(Chest circumference is body length): 2	Under 1 year- 9 to 13.5 2-3 years- 4 to 9 6-7 years- 0 to 4 818 years- 1 to 3
4	Life Index	The value of the vital capacity of the lungs (in ml) is divided by the body weight (in kg)	Husband: 60 Female: 50
5	Hand muscle strength	Hand strength (kg)*100 Weight(kg)	Male: 70% Female: 50%
6	Back muscle strength	Bench strength (kg)*100 Weight(kg)	Male: 220% Women: 135-150%
7	Fortress of Piñe's physique	D-(M+O) where D is the standing body length, M-body mass, O-chest circumference.	10-15 -sturdy 16-20 -good 21-25 -medium 26-30 - weak above 30 is very weak
8	Peizar	(Sitting body length): (Standing body length) x 100	In newborns, about 70 In adults, it's about 50
9	Verveca	(Body length) : (2 body weight + chest circumference)	1.35-1.25 - moderate predominance of growth in length 1.25-0.85 - harmonious development 0.85-0.75 - moderate brachymorphy.
10	Pirke index	Standing body length-sitting body lengthM00 Sitting body length	87%-small leg length, 87-92%-proportionate, over-92%-relatively long.

Appendix No. 2

Exercise scheme and a sample set of exercises for patients with asthenic chest and its deformities (funnel-shaped and keel-shaped degrees), training program

Class section	Objectives of the section	Lesson Content	Time
Part I introductory	Prepare all body systems for the main load	General-developing, breathing exercises (static and dynamic), quiet walking (simple and complicated).	7-10 min.
Part II - main part	Improved peripheral blood flow. Cardiorespiratory system training. Improvement of the psycho-emotional state of the patient. Increase in GIEF, strengthening of respiratory muscles. Strengthening the back muscles.	Starting position is sitting, lying on the back, on the stomach, standing on all fours, standing at the wall "Health" mode of medium loads at HR 110-130 per min. Work at the wall "Health" for 15 minutes. The number of approaches including 5-6 exercises for different muscle groups is individual and is determined by the pace of their performance. Exercise bikes.	30 min. 15 min.
III part- final	Reduce overall workload.	Breathing exercises, walking. In summer time - shower	5 min.

only 45 minutes

Appendix No. 3

Schematic of exercises in the physical therapy room for patients with posture disorders and scoliosis of I - III degree (group of people with low-explicit DST)

Class section	Objectives of the section	Lesson Content	Time
Part I introductory	Gradually prepare the body for the main load	Walking. Elementary general exercises for the upper and lower extremities. Breathing exercises.	5-7 min.
Part II - main part	Improving psycho emotional status. Strengthening the skill of correct posture. Formation of the "muscle corset". Improvement of the functional state of the heart and respiratory organs.	Mode of medium loads at HR 110-130 per min. General strengthening and specially corrective exercises (symmetrical and asymmetrical). I.p. - starting position lying on the back, stomach, side, kneeling, kneeling position. Dumbbells, benches, gymnastic wall, gymnastic sticks, balls are used in the classes.	30 min.
Part III - final	Reducing overall workload.	Statistical and dynamic relaxation breathing exercises, walking.	10 min.

only 45 minutes

Appendix No. 4

Scheme of therapeutic exercises for patients with severe DST

Class section	Objectives of the section	Lesson Content	Time
Part I introductory	Gradual activation of all organ systems. Preparing the respiratory and cardiac organs for high volume loads.	Walking. Dynamic and static breathing exercises. Elementary exercises for the muscles of the upper and lower extremities.	10 min.
Part II - main part	Activation of peripheral circulation. Improving psycho emotional state. Strengthening the respiratory muscles increase chest excursion. Improvement of metabolic processes in the myocardium.	Low-load mode at HR up to 110 min. General strengthening breathing exercises in various starting positions lying, sitting, standing. Inclusion of exercises with objects - gymnastic sticks, light dumbbells, balls, as well as exercises on a gymnastic wall and bench.	25 min.
Part III - final	Reduced workload.	Slow walking, relaxation exercises.	5 min.

only 45 minutes

Appendix No. 5

A set of special exercises for children with deformities of the BFD

Class section	Objectives of the section	Lesson Content	Time
Part I introductory	Improvement in the general condition of the patient. Improvement of psycho-emotional status of patients. Improving the conditions of blood supply and innervation of the BLA. Stimulation of reparative processes in damaged bone and soft tissues of the maxillofacial region.	Exercises for shoulder girdle muscles, upper limbs, dynamic breathing exercises. Rotations of the torso to the sides, alternate swinging movements of the lower limbs in different directions. Exercise for neck muscles: turns, bends and circular movements of the head.	2-3 min.
Part II - main part	Improvement and restoration of nasal breathing. Preventing the development of temporomandibular joint stiffness. Increased amplitude of movements in the TMJ. Strengthening of masticatory muscles, correction of lower jaw movements. Prevention of complications associated with hypokinesia and immobilization of the temporomandibular joint.	Exercises for mimic muscles, tongue muscles in combination with breathing through the nose. Exercise in sending impulses to the contraction of the masticatory muscles proper when the teeth are closed. Exercises for the muscles of the neck and upper limbs.	8-10 min.
Part III - final	Elimination of existing limitations in temporomandibular joint function.	Exercises in relaxing the muscles of the shoulder girdle, upper limbs and mimic muscles combined with deep breathing.	2-3 min.

12 to 16 minutes total

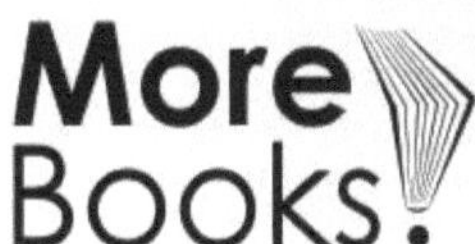

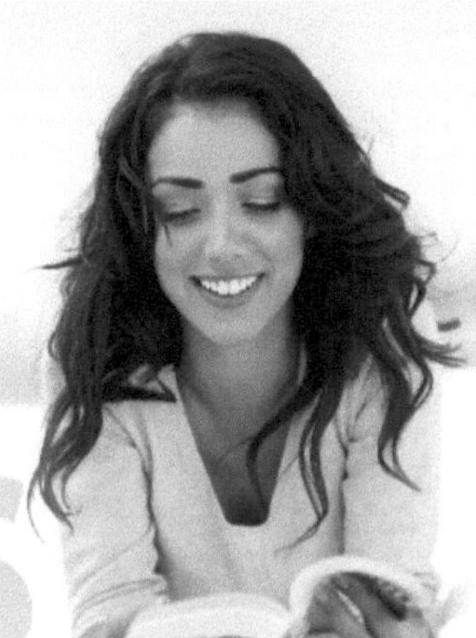

Buy your books fast and straightforward online - at one of world's fastest growing online book stores! Environmentally sound due to Print-on-Demand technologies.

Buy your books online at
www.morebooks.shop

Kaufen Sie Ihre Bücher schnell und unkompliziert online – auf einer der am schnellsten wachsenden Buchhandelsplattformen weltweit! Dank Print-On-Demand umwelt- und ressourcenschonend produziert.

Bücher schneller online kaufen
www.morebooks.shop

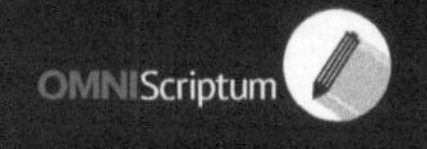

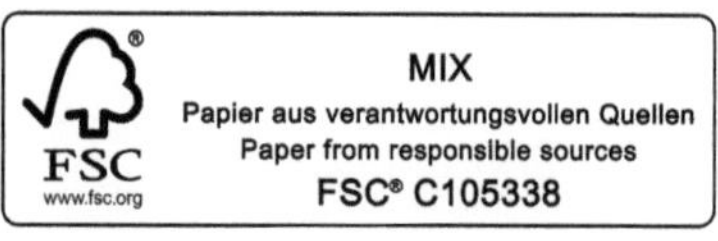

Printed by Books on Demand GmbH, Norderstedt / Germany